KETO COOKBOOK FOR BEGINNERS

Recipes For Quick &
Easy Low-Carb
Homemade Cooking

Diana Prince

TABLE OF CONTENTS

INTRODUCTION

Do you want to make a change in your life? Do you want to become a healthier person who can enjoy a new and improved life? Then, you are definitely in the right place. You are about to discover a wonderful and very healthy diet that has changed millions of lives. We are talking about the Ketogenic diet, a lifestyle that will mesmerize you and that will make you a new person in no time.

So, let's sit back, relax and find out more about the Ketogenic diet.

A keto diet is a low carb one. This is the first and one of the most important things you should now. During such a diet, your body makes ketones in your liver and these are used as energy.

Your body will produce less insulin and glucose and a state of ketosis is induced.

Ketosis is a natural process that appears when our food intake is lower than usual. The body will soon adapt to this state and therefore you will be able to lose weight in no time but you will also become healthier and your physical and mental performances will improve.

Your blood sugar levels will improve and you won't be predisposed to diabetes. Also, epilepsy and heart diseases can be prevented if you are on a Ketogenic diet. Your cholesterol will improve and you will feel amazing in no time.

How does that sound?

A Ketogenic diet is simple and easy to follow as long as you follow some simple rules. You don't need to make huge changes but there are some things you should know.

So, here goes!

BREAKFAST

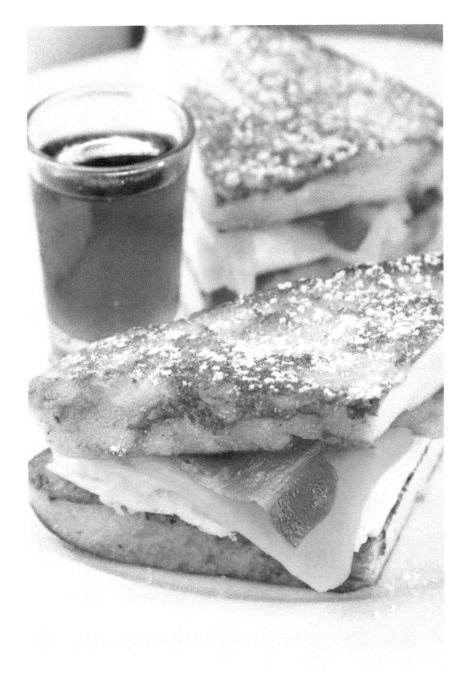

Avocado Muffins

If you like avocado recipes, then you should really try this next one soon!

Preparation time: 10 minutes **Cooking time:** 20 minutes **Servings:** 12

Ingredients:

4 eggs

6 bacon slices, chopped

1 yellow onion, chopped

1 cup coconut milk

2 cups avocado, pitted, peeled and chopped

Salt and black pepper to the taste

½ teaspoon baking soda

½ cup coconut flour

Directions:

1. Heat up a pan over medium heat, add onion and bacon, stir and brown for a few minutes.

2. In a bowl, mash avocado pieces with a fork and whisk well with the eggs.

3. Add milk, salt, pepper, baking soda and coconut flour and stir everything.

4. Add bacon mix and stir again.

5. Grease a muffin tray with the coconut oil, divide eggs and avocado mix into the tray, introduce in the oven at 350 degrees F and bake for 20 minutes.

6. Divide muffins between plates and serve them for breakfast. Enjoy!

Nutrition: calories 200, fat 7, fiber 4, carbs 7, protein 5

Bacon And Lemon Breakfast Muffins

We are sure you've never tried something like this before! It's a perfect keto breakfast!

Preparation time: 10 minutes **Cooking time:** 20 minutes **Servings:** 12

Ingredients:

1 cup bacon, finely chopped

Salt and black pepper to the taste

½ cup ghee, melted

3 cups almond flour

1 teaspoon baking soda

4 eggs

2 teaspoons lemon thyme

Directions:

1. In a bowl, mix flour with baking soda and eggs and stir well.

2. Add ghee, lemon thyme, bacon, salt and pepper and whisk well.

3. Divide this into a lined muffin pan, introduce in the oven at 350 degrees F and bake for 20 minutes.

4. Leave muffins to cool down a bit, divide between plates and serve them.

Enjoy!

Nutrition: calories 213, fat 7, fiber 2, carbs 9, protein 8

Cheese And Oregano Muffins

We will make you love keto muffins from now on!

Preparation time: 10 minutes **Cooking time:** 25 minutes **Servings:** 6

Ingredients:

2 tablespoons olive oil

1 egg

2 tablespoons parmesan cheese

½ teaspoon oregano, dried

1 cup almond flour

¼ teaspoon baking soda

Salt and black pepper to the taste

½ cup coconut milk

1 cup cheddar cheese, grated

Directions:

1. In a bowl, mix flour with oregano, salt, pepper, parmesan and baking soda and stir.

2. In another bowl, mix coconut milk with egg and olive oil and stir well.

3. Combine the 2 mixtures and whisk well.

4. Add cheddar cheese, stir, pour this a lined muffin tray, introduce in the oven at 350 degrees F for 25 minutes.

5. Leave your muffins to cool down for a few minutes, divide them between plates and serve.

Enjoy!

Nutrition: calories 160, fat 3, fiber 2, carbs 6, protein 10

Delicious Turkey Breakfast

Try a Ketogenic turkey breakfast for a change!

Preparation time: 10 minutes **Cooking time:** 20 minutes **Servings:** 1

Ingredients:

2 avocado slices

Salt and black pepper

2 bacon sliced

2 turkey breast slices, already cooked

2 tablespoons coconut oil

2 eggs, whisked

Directions:

1. Heat up a pan over medium heat, add bacon slices and brown them for a few minutes.

2. Meanwhile, heat up another pan with the oil over medium heat, add eggs, salt and pepper and scramble them.

3. Divide turkey breast slices on 2 plates.

4. Divide scrambled eggs on each.

5. Divide bacon slices and avocado slices as well and serve.

Enjoy!

Nutrition: calories 135, fat 7, fiber 2, carbs 4, protein 10

Amazing Burrito

Can you have a burrito for breakfast? Of course, you can!

Preparation time: 10 minutes **Cooking time:** 16 minutes **Servings:** 1

Ingredients:

1 teaspoon coconut oil

1 teaspoon garlic powder

1 teaspoon cumin, ground

¼ pound beef meat, ground

1 teaspoon sweet paprika

1 teaspoon onion powder

1 small red onion, julienned

1 teaspoon cilantro, chopped

Salt and black pepper to the taste

3 eggs

Directions:

1. Heat up a pan over medium heat, add beef and brown for a few minutes.

2. Add salt, pepper, cumin, garlic and onion powder and paprika, stir, cook for 4 minutes more and take off heat.

3. In a bowl, mix eggs with salt and pepper and whisk well.

4. Heat up a pan with the oil over medium heat, add egg, spread evenly and cook for 6 minutes.

5. Transfer your egg burrito to a plate, divide beef mix, add onion and cilantro, roll and serve.

Enjoy!

Nutrition: calories 280, fat 12, fiber 4, carbs 7, protein 14

Amazing Breakfast Hash

This breakfast hash is just right for you!

Preparation time: 10 minutes **Cooking time:** 16 minutes **Servings:** 2

Ingredients:

1 tablespoon coconut oil

2 garlic cloves, minced

½ cup beef stock

Salt and black pepper to the taste

1 yellow onion, chopped

2 cups corned beef, chopped

1 pound radishes, cut in quarters

Directions:

1. Heat up a pan with the oil over medium high heat, add onion, stir and cook for 4 minutes.

2. Add radishes, stir and cook for 5 minutes.

3. Add garlic, stir and cook for 1 minute more.

4. Add stock, beef, salt and pepper, stir, cook for 5 minutes, take off heat and serve.

Enjoy!

Nutrition: calories 240, fat 7, fiber 3, carbs 12, protein 8

Brussels Sprouts Delight

This is so tasty and very easy to make! It's a great keto breakfast idea for you!

Preparation time: 10 minutes **Cooking time:** 12 minutes **Servings:** 3

Ingredients:

3 eggs

Salt and black pepper to the taste

1 tablespoon ghee, melted

2 shallots, minced

2 garlic cloves, minced

12 ounces Brussels sprouts, thinly sliced

2 ounces bacon, chopped

1 and ½ tablespoons apple cider vinegar

Directions:

1. Heat up a pan over medium heat, add bacon, stir, cook until it's crispy, transfer to a plate and leave aside for now.

2. Heat up the pan again over medium heat, add shallots and garlic, stir and cook for 30 seconds.

3. Add Brussels sprouts, salt, pepper and apple cider vinegar, stir and cook for 5 minutes.

4. Return bacon to pan, stir and cook for 5 minutes more.

5. Add ghee, stir and make a hole in the center.

6. Crack eggs into the pan, cook until they are done and serve right away.

Enjoy!

Nutrition: calories 240, fat 7, fiber 4, carbs 7, protein 12

Breakfast Cereal Nibs

Pay attention and learn how to prepare the best keto cereal nibs!

Preparation time: 10 minutes **Cooking time:** 45minutes **Servings:** 4

Ingredients:

4 tablespoons hemp hearts

½ cup chia seeds

1 cup water

1 tablespoon vanilla extract

1 tablespoon psyllium powder

2 tablespoons coconut oil

1 tablespoon swerve

2 tablespoons cocoa nibs

Directions:

1. In a bowl, mix chia seeds with water, stir and leave aside for 5 minutes.

2. Add hemp hearts, vanilla extract, psyllium powder, oil and swerve and stir well with your mixer.

3. Add cocoa nibs, and stir until you obtain a dough.

4. Divide dough into 2 pieces, shape into cylinder form, place on a lined baking sheet, flatten well, cover with a parchment paper, introduce in the oven at 285 degrees F and bake for 20 minutes.

5. Remove the parchment paper and bake for 25 minutes more.

6. Take cylinders out of the oven, leave aside to cool down and cut into small pieces.

7. Serve in the morning with some almond milk.

Enjoy!

Nutrition: calories 245, fat 12, fiber 12, carbs 2, protein 9

Breakfast Chia Pudding

Try a chia pudding this morning!

Preparation time: 10 minutes **Cooking time:** 30 minutes **Servings:** 2

Ingredients:

2 tablespoons coffee

2 cups water

1/3 cup chia seeds

1 tablespoon swerve

1 tablespoon vanilla extract

2 tablespoons cocoa nibs

1/3 cup coconut cream

Directions:

1. Heat up a small pot with the water over medium heat, bring to a boil, add coffee, simmer for 15 minutes, take off heat and strain into a bowl.

2. Add vanilla extract, coconut cream, swerve, cocoa nibs and chia seeds, stir well, keep in the fridge for 30 minutes, divide into 2 breakfast bowls and serve.

Enjoy!

Nutrition: calories 100, fat 0.4, fiber 4, carbs 3, protein 3

Delicious Hemp Porridge

It's a hearty and 100% keto breakfast idea!

Preparation time: 3 minutes **Cooking time:** 3 minutes **Servings:** 1

Ingredients:

1 tablespoon chia seeds

1 cup almond milk

2 tablespoons flax seeds

½ cup hemp hearts

½ teaspoon cinnamon, ground

1 tablespoon stevia

¾ teaspoon vanilla extract

¼ cup almond flour

1 tablespoon hemp hearts for serving

Directions:

1. In a pan, mix almond milk with ½ cup hemp hearts, chia seeds, stevia, flax seeds, cinnamon and vanilla extract, stir well and heat up over medium heat.

2. Cook for 2 minutes, take off heat, add almond flour, stir well and pour into a bowl.

3. Top with 1 tablespoon hemp hearts and serve.

Enjoy!

Nutrition: calories 230, fat 12, fiber 7, carbs 3, protein 43

LUNCH

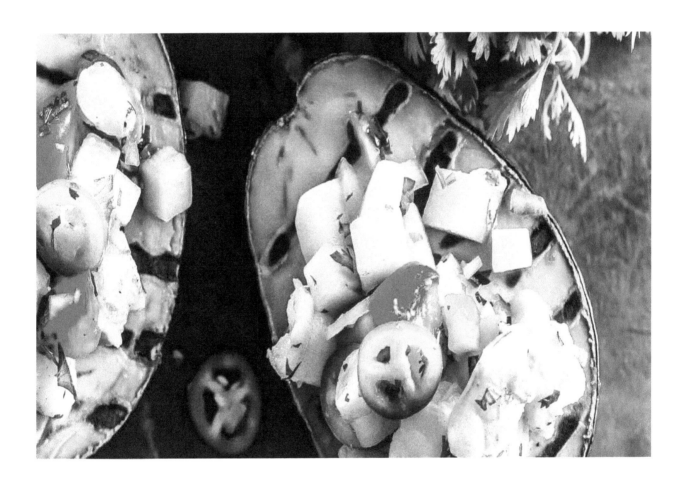

Pumpkin Soup

This keto soup is very creamy and textured! You should really try it for lunch today!

Preparation time: 10 minutes **Cooking time:** 20 minutes **Servings:** 6

Ingredients:½ cup yellow onion, chopped

2 tablespoons olive oil

1 tablespoon chipotles in adobo sauce

1 garlic clove, minced

1 teaspoon cumin, ground

1 teaspoon coriander, ground

A pinch of allspice

2 cups pumpkin puree

Salt and black pepper to the taste

32 ounces chicken stock

½ cup heavy cream

2 teaspoons vinegar

2 teaspoons stevia

Directions:

1. Heat up a pot with the oil over medium heat, add onions and garlic, stir and cook for 4 minutes.

2. Add stevia, cumin, coriander, chipotles and cumin, stir and cook for 2 minutes.

3. Add stock and pumpkin puree, stir and cook for 5 minutes.

4. Blend soup well using an immersion blender and then mix with salt, pepper, heavy cream and vinegar.

5. Stir, cook for 5 minutes more and divide into bowls.

6. Serve right away.

Enjoy!

Nutrition: calories 140, fat 12, fiber 3, carbs 6, protein 2

Delicious Green Beans Casserole

This will impress you for sure!

Preparation time: 10 minutes **Cooking time:** 35 minutes **Servings:** 8

Ingredients:

1 pound green beans, halved

Salt and black pepper to the taste

½ cup almond flour

2 tablespoons ghee

8 ounces mushrooms, chopped

4 ounces onion, chopped

2 shallots, chopped

3 garlic cloves, minced

½ cup chicken stock

½ cup heavy cream

¼ cup parmesan, grated

Avocado oil for frying

Directions:

1. Put some water in a pot, add salt, bring to a boil over medium high heat, add green beans, cook for 5 minutes, transfer to a bowl filled with ice water, cool down, drain well and leave aside for now.

2. In a bowl, mix shallots with onions, almond flour, salt and pepper and toss to coat.

3. Heat up a pan with some avocado oil over medium high heat, add onions and shallots mix, fry until they are golden.

4. Transfer to paper towels and drain grease.

5. Heat up the same pan over medium heat, add ghee and melt it.

6. Add garlic and mushrooms, stir and cook for 5 minutes.

7. Add stock and heavy cream, stir, bring to a boil and simmer until it thickens.

8. Add parmesan and green beans, toss to coat and take off heat.

9. Transfer this mix to a baking dish, sprinkle crispy onions mix all over, introduce in the oven at 400 degrees F and bake for 15 minutes.

10. Serve warm.

Enjoy!

Nutrition: calories 155, fat, 11, fiber 6, carbs 8, protein 5

Simple Lunch Apple Salad

This is not just Ketogenic! It's also very tasty!

Preparation time: 10 minutes **Cooking time:** 0 minutes **Servings:** 4

Ingredients:

2 cups broccoli florets, roughly chopped

2 ounces pecans, chopped

1 apple, cored and grated

1 green onion stalk, finely chopped

Salt and black pepper to the taste

2 teaspoons poppy seeds

1 teaspoon apple cider vinegar

¼ cup mayonnaise

½ teaspoon lemon juice

¼ cup sour cream

Directions:

1. In a salad bowl, mix apple with broccoli, green onion and pecans and stir.

2. Add poppy seeds, salt and pepper and toss gently.

3. In a bowl, mix mayo with sour cream, vinegar and lemon juice and whisk well.

4. Pour this over salad, toss to coat well and serve cold for lunch! Enjoy!

Nutrition: calories 250, fat 23, fiber 4, carbs 4, protein 5

Brussels Sprouts Gratin

It's a dense and rich keto lunch idea!

Preparation time: 10 minutes **Cooking time:** 35 minutes **Servings:** 4
Ingredients:

2 ounces onions, chopped

1 teaspoon garlic, minced

6 ounces Brussels sprouts, chopped

2 tablespoons ghee

1 tablespoon coconut aminos

Salt and black pepper to the taste

½ teaspoon liquid smoke

For the sauce:

2.5 ounces cheddar cheese, grated

A pinch of black pepper

1 tablespoon ghee

½ cup heavy cream

¼ teaspoon turmeric

¼ teaspoon paprika

A pinch of xanthan gum

For the pork crust:

3 tablespoons parmesan

0.5 ounces pork rinds

½ teaspoon sweet paprika

Directions:

1. Heat up a pan with 2 tablespoons ghee over high heat, add Brussels sprouts, salt and pepper, stir and cook for 3 minutes.

2. Add garlic and onion, stir and cook for 3 minutes more.

3. Add liquid smoke and coconut aminos, stir, take off heat and

leave aside for now.

4. Heat up another pan with 1 tablespoon ghee over medium heat, add heavy cream and stir.

5. Add cheese, black pepper, turmeric, paprika and xanthan gum, stir and cook until it thickens again.

6. Add Brussels sprouts mix, toss to coat and divide into ramekins.

7. In your food processor, mix parmesan with pork rinds and ½ teaspoon paprika and pulse well.

8. Divide these crumbs on top of Brussels sprouts mix, introduce ramekins in the oven at 375 degrees F and bake for 20 minutes.

9. Serve right away.

Enjoy!

Nutrition: calories 300, fat 20, fiber 6, carbs 5, protein 10

Simple Asparagus Lunch

You only need a few ingredients and a few minutes of your time to make this simple and very tasty keto lunch!

Preparation time: 10 minutes **Cooking time:** 10 minutes **Servings:** 4

Ingredients:

2 egg yolks

Salt and black pepper to the taste

¼ cup ghee

1 tablespoon lemon juice

A pinch of cayenne pepper

40 asparagus spears

Directions:

1. In a bowl, whisk egg yolks very well.

2. Transfer this to a small pan over low heat.

3. Add lemon juice and whisk well.

4. Add ghee and whisk until it melts.

5. Add salt, pepper and cayenne pepper and whisk again well.

6. Meanwhile, heat up a pan over medium high heat, add asparagus spears and fry them for 5 minutes.

7. Divide asparagus on plates, drizzle the sauce you've made on top and serve.

Enjoy!

Nutrition: calories 150, fat 13, fiber 6, carbs 2, protein 3

Simple Shrimp Pasta

This is so yummy!

Preparation time: 10 minutes **Cooking time:** 10 minutes **Servings:** 4

Ingredients:

12 ounces angel hair noodles

2 tablespoons olive oil

Salt and black pepper to the taste

2 tablespoons ghee

4 garlic cloves, minced

1 pound shrimp, raw, peeled and deveined

Juice of ½ lemon

½ teaspoon paprika

A handful basil, chopped

Directions:

1. Put water in a pot, add some salt, bring to a boil, add noodles, cook for 2 minutes, drain them and transfer to a heated pan.

2. Toast noodles for a few seconds, take off heat and leave them aside.

3. Heat up a pan with the ghee and olive oil over medium heat, add garlic, stir and brown for 1 minute.

4. Add shrimp and lemon juice and cook for 3 minutes on each side.

5. Add noodles, salt, pepper and paprika, stir, divide into bowls and serve with chopped basil on top.

Enjoy!

Nutrition: calories 300, fat 20, fiber 6, carbs 3, protein 30

Incredible Mexican Casserole

Try this Mexican Ketogenic lunch will surprise you for sure!

Preparation time: 10 minutes **Cooking time:** 35 minutes **Servings:** 6

Ingredients:

2 chipotle peppers, chopped

2 jalapenos, chopped

1 tablespoon olive oil

¼ cup heavy cream

1 small white onion, chopped

Salt and black pepper to the taste

1 pound chicken thighs, skinless, boneless and chopped

1 cup red enchilada sauce

4 ounces cream cheese

Cooking spray

1 cup pepper jack cheese, shredded

2 tablespoons cilantro, chopped

2 tortillas

Directions:

1. Heat up a pan with the oil over medium heat, add chipotle and jalapeno peppers, stir and cook for a few seconds.

2. Add onion, stir and cook for 5 minutes.

3. Add cream cheese and heavy cream and stir until cheese melts.

4. Add chicken, salt, pepper and enchilada sauce, stir well and take off heat.

5. Grease a baking dish with cooking spray, place tortillas on the bottom, spread chicken mix all over and sprinkle shredded cheese.

6. Cover with tin foil, introduce in the oven at 350 degrees F and bake for 15 minutes.

7. Remove the tin foil and bake for 15 minutes more.

8. Sprinkle cilantro on top and serve.

Enjoy!

Nutrition: calories 240, fat 12, fiber 5, carbs 5, protein 20

Delicious Asian Lunch Salad

Try this exotic lunch salad tomorrow!

Preparation time: 10 minutes **Cooking time:** 15 minutes **Servings:** 4

Ingredients:

1 pound beef, ground

1 tablespoon sriracha

2 tablespoons coconut aminos

2 garlic cloves, minced

10 ounces coleslaw mix

2 tablespoon sesame seed oil

Salt and black pepper to the taste

1 teaspoon apple cider vinegar

1 teaspoon sesame seeds

1 green onion stalk, chopped

Directions:

1. Heat up a pan with the oil over medium heat, add garlic and brown for 1 minute.

2. Add beef, stir and cook for 10 minutes.

3. Add cole slaw mix, toss to coat and cook for 1minute.

4. Add vinegar, sriracha, coconut aminos, salt and pepper, stir and cook for 4 minutes more.

5. Add green onions and sesame seeds, toss to coat, divide into bowls and serve for lunch.

Enjoy!

Nutrition: calories 350, fat 23, fiber 6, carbs 3, protein 20

Simple Buffalo Wings

You must try these for lunch if you are on a keto diet!

Preparation time: 10 minutes **Cooking time:** 20 minutes **Servings:** 2

Ingredients:

2 tablespoons ghee

6 chicken wings, cut in halves

Salt and black pepper to the taste

A pinch of garlic powder

½ cup hot sauce

A pinch of cayenne pepper

½ teaspoon sweet paprika

Directions:

1. In a bowl, mix chicken pieces with half of the hot sauce, salt and pepper and toss well to coat.

2. Arrange chicken pieces on a lined baking dish, introduce in preheated broiler and broil 8 minutes.

3. Flip chicken pieces and broil for 8 minutes more.

4. Heat up a pan with the ghee over medium heat.

5. Add the rest of the hot sauce, salt, pepper, cayenne and paprika, stir and cook for a couple of minutes.

6. Transfer broiled chicken pieces to a bowl, add ghee and hot sauce mix over them and toss to coat well.

7. Serve them right away!

Enjoy!

Nutrition: calories 500, fat 45, fiber 12, carbs 1, protein 45

Amazing Bacon And Mushrooms Skewers

You only need about 20 minutes to make this simple and very tasty lunch!

Preparation time: 10 minutes **Cooking time:** 20 minutes **Servings:** 6

Ingredients:

1 pound mushroom caps

6 bacon strips

Salt and black pepper to the taste

½ teaspoon sweet paprika

Some sweet mesquite

Directions:

1. Season mushroom caps with salt, pepper and paprika.

2. Spear a bacon strip on a skewer's ends.

3. Spear a mushroom cap and fold over bacon.

4. Repeat until you obtain a mushroom and bacon braid.

5. Repeat with the rest of the mushrooms and bacon strip.

6. Season with sweet mesquite, place all skewers on preheated kitchen grill over medium heat, cook for 10 minutes, flip and cook for 10 minutes more.

7. Divide between plates and serve for lunch with a side salad! Enjoy!

Nutrition: calories 110, fat 7, fiber 4, carbs 2, protein 10

SIDE DISH

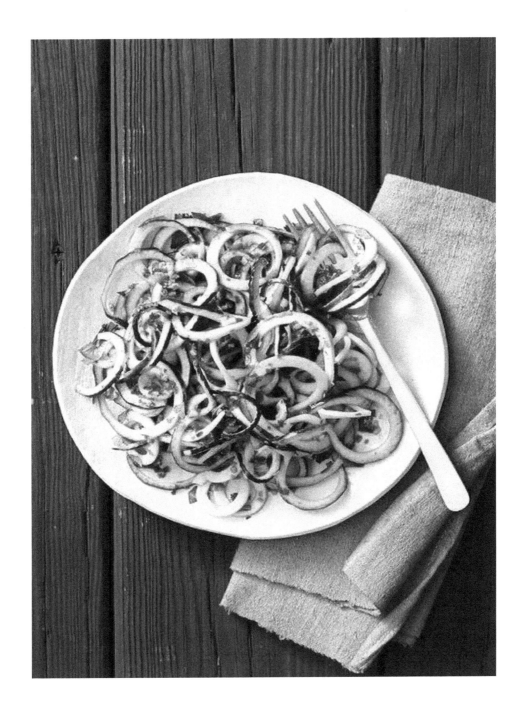

Indian Mint Chutney

It has such a unique color and taste! It's a special side for any steak!

Preparation time: 10 minutes **Cooking time:** 0 minutes **Servings:** 8

Ingredients:

1 and ½ cup mint leaves

1 big bunch cilantro

Salt and black pepper to the taste

1 green chili pepper, seedless

1 yellow onion, cut into medium chunks

¼ cup water

1 tablespoon tamarind juice

Directions:

1. Put mint and coriander leaves in your food processor and blend them.

2. Add chili pepper, salt, black pepper, onion and tamarind paste and blend again.

3. Add water, blend some more until you obtain cream, transfer to a bowl and serve as a side for a tasty keto steak.

Enjoy!

Nutrition: calories 100, fat 1, fiber 1, carbs 0.4, protein 6

Indian Coconut Chutney

It's perfect for a fancy Indian style Ketogenic dish!

Preparation time: 5 minutes **Cooking time:** 5 minutes **Servings:** 3

Ingredients: ½ teaspoon cumin

½ cup coconut, grated

2 tablespoons already fried chana dal

2 green chilies

Salt to the taste

1 garlic clove

¾ tablespoons avocado oil

¼ teaspoon mustard seeds

A pinch of hing

½ teaspoons urad dal

1 red chili chopped

1 spring curry leaves

Directions:

1. In your food processor, mix coconut with salt to the taste, cumin, garlic, chana dal and green chilies and blend well.

2. Add a splash of water and blend again.

3. Heat up a pan with the oil over medium heat, add red chili, urad dal, mustard seeds, hing and curry leaves, stir and cook for 2-3 minutes.

4. Add this to coconut chutney, stir gently and serve as a side.

Enjoy!

Nutrition: calories 90, fat 1, fiber 1, carbs 1, protein 6

Easy Tamarind Chutney

It's sweet and it's perfectly balanced! It's one of the best sides for a keto dish!

Preparation time: 10 minutes **Cooking time:** 35 minutes **Servings:** 10

Ingredients:

1 teaspoon cumin seeds

1 tablespoon canola oil

½ teaspoon garam masala

½ teaspoon asafetida powder

1 teaspoon ground ginger

½ teaspoon fennel seeds

½ teaspoon cayenne pepper

1 and ¼ cups coconut sugar

2 cups water

3 tablespoons tamarind paste

Directions:

1. Heat up a pan with the oil over medium heat, add ginger, cumin, cayenne pepper, asafetida powder, fennel seeds and garam masala, stir and cook for 2 minutes.

2. Add water, sugar and tamarind paste, stir, bring to a boil, reduce heat

to low and simmer chutney for 30 minutes.

3. Transfer to a bowl and leave it to cool down before you serve it as a side for a steak.

Enjoy!

Nutrition: calories 120, fat 1, fiber 3, carbs 5, protein 9

Caramelized Bell Peppers

A Ketogenic pork dish will taste much better with such a side dish!

Preparation time: 10 minutes **Cooking time:** 32 minutes **Servings:** 4
Ingredients:

1 tablespoon olive oil

1 teaspoon ghee

2 red bell peppers, cut into thin strips

2 red onions, cut into thin strips

Salt and black pepper to the taste

1 teaspoon basil, dried

Directions:

1. Heat up a pan with the ghee and the oil over medium heat, add onion and bell peppers, stir and cook for 2 minutes.

2. Reduce temperature and cook for 30 minutes more stirring often.

3. Add salt, pepper and basil, stir again, take off heat and serve as a keto side dish.

Enjoy!

Nutrition: calories 97, fat 4, fiber 2, carbs 6, protein 2

Caramelized Red Chard

This is an easy side for a dinner dish!

Preparation time: 10 minutes **Cooking time:** 20 minutes **Servings:** 4

Ingredients:

2 tablespoons olive oil

1 yellow onion, chopped

2 tablespoons capers

Juice of 1 lemon

Salt and black pepper to the taste

1 teaspoon palm sugar

1 bunch red chard, chopped

¼ cup kalamata olives, pitted and chopped

Directions:

1. Heat up a pan with the oil over medium heat, add onions, stir and brown for 4 minutes.

2. Add palm sugar and stir well.

3. Add olives and chard, stir and cook for 10 minutes more.

4. Add capers, lemon juice, salt and pepper, stir and cook for 3 minutes more.

5. Divide between plates and serve as a keto side.

Enjoy!

Nutrition: calories 119, fat 7, fiber 3, carbs 7, protein 2

Special Summer Kale Side Dish

This is perfect as a keto side dish for a summer delight!

Preparation time: 10 minutes **Cooking time:** 45 minutes **Servings:** 4

Ingredients:

2 cups water

1 tablespoon balsamic vinegar

1/3 cup almonds, toasted

3 garlic cloves, minced

1 bunch kale, steamed and chopped

1 small yellow onion, chopped

2 tablespoons olive oil

Directions:

1. Heat up a pan with the oil over medium heat, add onion, stir and cook for 10 minutes.

2. Add garlic, stir and cook for 1 minute.

3. Add water and kale, cover pan and cook for 30 minutes.

4. Add salt, pepper, balsamic vinegar and almonds, toss to coat, divide between plates and serve as a side.

Enjoy!

Nutrition: calories 170, fat 11, fiber 3, carbs 7, protein 7

Amazing Coleslaw

Coleslaws are very famous! Today, we recommend you a keto one!

Preparation time: 10 minutes **Cooking time:** 0 minutes **Servings:** 4

Ingredients:

1 small green cabbage head, shredded

Salt and black pepper to the taste

6 tablespoons mayonnaise

Salt and black pepper to the taste

1 pinch fennel seed

Juice of ½ lemon

1 tablespoon Dijon mustard

Directions:

1. In a bowl, mix cabbage with salt and lemon juice, stir well and leave aside for 10 minutes.

2. Press well the cabbage, add more salt and pepper, fennel seed, mayo and mustard.

3. Toss to coat and serve.

Enjoy!

Nutrition: calories 150, fat 3, fiber 2, carbs 2, protein 7

Simple Fried Cabbage

The cabbage is such a versatile veggie! Try this amazing side dish as soon as possible!

Preparation time: 10 minutes **Cooking time:** 15 minutes **Servings:** 4

Ingredients:

1 and ½ pound green cabbage, shredded

Salt and black pepper to the taste

3.5 ounces ghee

A pinch of sweet paprika

Directions:

1. Heat up a pan with the ghee over medium heat.

2. Add cabbage and cook for 15 minutes stirring often.

3. Add salt, pepper and paprika, stir, cook for 1 minute more, divide between plates and serve.

Enjoy!

Nutrition: calories 200, fat 4, fiber 2, carbs 3, protein 7

Delicious Green Beans And Avocado

Serve this with a tasty fish dish!

Preparation time: 10 minutes **Cooking time:** 5 minutes **Servings:** 4

Ingredients:

2/3 pound green beans, trimmed

Salt and black pepper to the taste

3 tablespoons olive oil

2 avocados, pitted and peeled

5 scallions, chopped

A handful cilantro, chopped

Directions:

1. Heat up a pan with the oil over medium heat, add green beans, stir and cook for 4 minutes.

2. Add salt and pepper, stir, take off heat and transfer to a bowl.

3. In another bowl, mix avocados with salt and pepper and mash with a fork.

4. Add onions and stir well.

5. Add this over green beans, toss to coat and serve with chopped cilantro on top.

Enjoy!

Nutrition: calories 200, fat 5, fiber 3, carbs 4, protein 6

Creamy Spaghetti Pasta

This is just perfect for a turkey dish!

Preparation time: 10 minutes **Cooking time:** 40 minutes **Servings:** 4

Ingredients:

1 spaghetti squash

Salt and black pepper to the taste

2 tablespoons ghee

1 teaspoon Cajun seasoning

A pinch of cayenne pepper

2 cups heavy cream

Directions:

1. Prick spaghetti with a fork, place on a lined baking sheet, introduce in the oven at 350 degrees F and bake for 15 minutes.

2. Take spaghetti squash out of the oven, leave aside to cool down a bit

and scoop squash noodles.

3. Heat up a pan with the ghee over medium heat, add spaghetti squash,

stir and cook for a couple of minutes.

4. Add salt, pepper, cayenne pepper and Cajun seasoning, stir and cook

for 1 minute.

5. Add heavy cream, stir, cook for 10 minutes more, divide between plates and serve as a keto side dish.

Enjoy!

Nutrition: calories 200, fat 2, fiber 1, carbs 5, protein 8

APPETIZERS

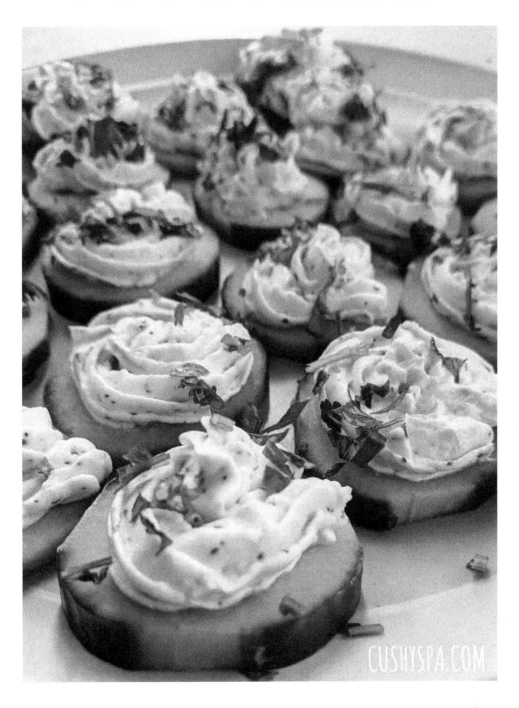

Almond Butter Bars

This is a great keto snack for a casual day!

Preparation time: 2 hours and 10 minutes **Cooking time:** 2 minutes
Servings:

12

Ingredients: ¾ cup coconut, unsweetened and shredded

¾ cup almond butter

¾ cup stevia

1 cup almond butter

2 tablespoons almond butter

4.5 ounces dark chocolate, chopped

2 tablespoons coconut oil

Directions:

1. In a bowl, mix almond flour with stevia and coconut and stir well.

2. Heat up a pan over medium-low heat, add 1 cup almond butter and the coconut oil and whisk well.

3. Add this to almond flour and stir well.

4. Transfer this to a baking dish and press well.

5. Heat up another pan with the chocolate stirring often.

6. Add the rest of the almond butter and whisk well again.

7. Pour this over almond mix and spread evenly.

8. Introduce in the fridge for 2 hours, cut into 12 bars and serve as a keto snack.

Enjoy!

Nutrition: calories 140, fat 2, fiber 1, carbs 5, protein 1

Tasty Zucchini Snack

Try this today!

Preparation time: 10 minutes **Cooking time:** 15 minutes **Servings:** 4

Ingredients:

1 cup mozzarella, shredded

¼ cup tomato sauce

1 zucchini, sliced

Salt and black pepper to the taste

A pinch of cumin

Cooking spray

Directions:

1. Spray a cooking sheet with some oil and arrange zucchini slices.

2. Spread tomato sauce all over zucchini slices, season with salt, pepper and cumin and sprinkle shredded mozzarella.

3. Introduce in the oven at 350 degrees F and bake for 15 minutes.

4. Arrange on a platter and serve.

Enjoy!

Nutrition: calories 140, fat 4, fiber 2, carbs 6, protein 4

Zucchini Chips

Enjoy a great snack with only a few calories!

Preparation time: 10 minutes **Cooking time:** 3 hours **Servings:** 8

Ingredients:

3 zucchinis, very thinly sliced

Salt and black pepper to the taste

2 tablespoons olive oil

2 tablespoons balsamic vinegar

Directions:

1. In a bowl, mix oil with vinegar, salt and pepper and whisk well.

2. Add zucchini slices, toss to coat well and spread on a lined baking sheet, introduce in the oven at 200 degrees F and bake for 3 hours.

3. Leave chips to cool down and serve them as a keto snack. Enjoy!

Nutrition: calories 40, fat 3, fiber 7, carbs 3, protein 7

Simple Hummus

Everyone loves a good hummus! Try this one!

Preparation time: 10 minutes **Cooking time:** 0 minutes **Servings:** 5

Ingredients:

4 cups zucchinis, finely chopped

¼ cup olive oil

Salt and black pepper to the taste

4 garlic cloves, minced

¾ cup tahini

½ cup lemon juice

1 tablespoon cumin, ground

Directions:

1. In your blender, mix zucchinis with salt, pepper, oil, lemon juice, garlic, tahini and cumin and blend very well.

2. Transfer to a bowl and serve.

Enjoy!

Nutrition: calories 80, fat 5, fiber 3, carbs 6, protein 7

Amazing Celery Sticks

This is so great! It's an amazing keto snack, indeed!

Preparation time: 10 minutes **Cooking time:** 0 minutes **Servings:** 12

Ingredients:

2 cups rotisserie chicken, shredded

6 celery sticks cut in halves

3 tablespoons hot tomato sauce

¼ cup mayonnaise

Salt and black pepper to the taste

½ teaspoon garlic powder

Some chopped chives for serving

Directions:

1. In a bowl, mix chicken with salt, pepper, garlic powder, mayo and tomato sauce and stir well.

2. Arrange celery pieces on a platter, spread chicken mix over them, sprinkle some chives and serve.

Enjoy!

Nutrition: calories 100, fat 2, fiber 3, carbs 1, protein 6

Beef Jerky Snack

We are sure you will love this keto snack!

Preparation time: 6 hours **Cooking time:** 4 hours **Servings:** 6

Ingredients:

24 ounces amber

2 cups soy sauce

½ cup Worcestershire sauce

2 tablespoons black peppercorns

2 tablespoons black pepper

2 pounds beef round, sliced

Directions:

1. In a bowl, mix soy sauce with black peppercorns, black pepper and Worcestershire sauce and whisk well.

2. Add beef slices, toss to coat and leave aside in the fridge for 6 hours.

3. Spread this on a rack, introduce in the oven at 370 degrees F and bake for 4 hours.

4. Transfer to a bowl and serve.

Enjoy!

Nutrition: calories 300, fat 12, fiber 4, carbs 3, protein 8

Crab Dip

You will adore this amazing keto appetizer!

Preparation time: 10 minutes **Cooking time:** 30 minutes **Servings:** 8

Ingredients:

8 bacon strips, sliced

12 ounces crab meat

½ cup mayonnaise

½ cup sour cream

8 ounces cream cheese

2 poblano pepper, chopped

2 tablespoons lemon juice

Salt and black pepper to the taste

4 garlic cloves, minced

4 green onions, minced

½ cup parmesan cheese+ ½ cup parmesan cheese, grated

Salt and black pepper to the taste

Directions:

1. Heat up a pan over medium high heat, add bacon, cook until it's crispy, transfer to paper towels, chop and leave aside to cool down.

2. In a bowl, mix sour cream with cream cheese and mayo and stir well.

3. Add ½ cup parmesan, poblano peppers, bacon, green onion, garlic and lemon juice and stir again.

4. Add crab meat, salt and pepper and stir gently.

5. Pour this into a heatproof baking dish, spread the rest of the parm, introduce in the oven and bake at 350 degrees F for 20

minutes.

6. Serve your dip warm with cucumber stick.

Enjoy!

Nutrition: calories 200, fat 7, fiber 2, carbs 4, protein 6

Simple Spinach Balls

This is a very tasty keto party appetizer!

Preparation time: 10 minutes **Cooking time:** 12 minutes **Servings:** 30

Ingredients:

4 tablespoons melted ghee

2 eggs

1 cup almond flour

16 ounces spinach

1/3 cup feta cheese, crumbled

¼ teaspoon nutmeg, ground

1/3 cup parmesan, grated

Salt and black pepper to the taste

1 tablespoon onion powder

3 tablespoons whipping cream

1 teaspoon garlic powder

Directions:

1. In your blender, mix spinach with ghee, eggs, almond flour, feta cheese, parmesan, nutmeg, whipping cream, salt, pepper, onion and garlic pepper and blend very well.

2. Transfer to a bowl and keep in the freezer for 10 minutes

3. Shape 30 spinach balls, arrange on a lined baking sheet, introduce in the oven at 350 degrees F and bake for 12 minutes.

4. Leave spinach balls to cool down and serve as a party appetizer.

Enjoy!

Nutrition: calories 60, fat 5, fiber 1, carbs 0.7, protein 2

Garlic Spinach Dip

This keto appetizer will make you love spinach even more!

Preparation time: 10 minutes **Cooking time:** 35 minutes **Servings:** 6

Ingredients:

6 bacon slices

5 ounces spinach

½ cup sour cream

8 ounces cream cheese, soft

1 and ½ tablespoons parsley, chopped

2.5 ounces parmesan, grated

1 tablespoon lemon juice

Salt and black pepper to the taste

1 tablespoon garlic, minced

Directions:

1. Heat up a pan over medium heat, add bacon, cook until it's crispy, transfer to paper towels, drain grease, crumble and leave aside in a bowl.

2. Heat up the same pan with the bacon grease over medium heat, add spinach, stir, cook for 2 minutes and transfer to a bowl.

3. In another bowl, mix cream cheese with garlic, salt, pepper, sour cream and parsley and stir well.

4. Add bacon and stir again.

5. Add lemon juice and spinach and stir everything.

6. Add parmesan and stir again.

7. Divide this into ramekins, introduce in the oven at 350 degrees f and bake for 25 minutes.

8. Turn oven to broil and broil for 4 minutes more.

9. Serve with crackers.

Enjoy!

Nutrition: calories 345, fat 12, fiber 3, carbs 6, protein 11

Mushrooms Appetizer

These mushrooms are so yummy!

Preparation time: 10 minutes **Cooking time:** 20 minutes **Servings:** 5

Ingredients:¼ cup mayo

1 teaspoon garlic powder

1 small yellow onion, chopped

24 ounces white mushroom caps

Salt and black pepper to the taste

1 teaspoon curry powder

4 ounces cream cheese, soft

¼ cup sour cream

½ cup Mexican cheese, shredded

1 cup shrimp, cooked, peeled, deveined and chopped

Directions:

1. In a bowl, mix mayo with garlic powder, onion, curry powder, cream cheese, sour cream, Mexican cheese, shrimp, salt and pepper to the taste and whisk well.

2. Stuff mushrooms with this mix, place on a baking sheet and cook in the oven at 350 degrees F for 20 minutes.

3. Arrange on a platter and serve.

Enjoy!

Nutrition: calories 244, fat 20, fiber 3, carbs 7, protein 14

VEGETABLE

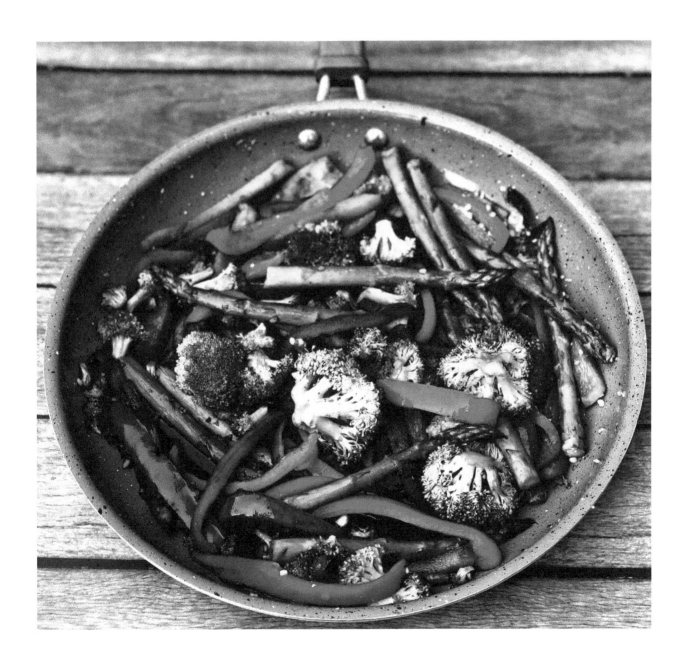

Amazing Broccoli And Cauliflower Cream

This is so textured and delicious!

Preparation time: 10 minutes **Cooking time:** 15 minutes **Servings:** 5

Ingredients:

1 cauliflower head, florets separated

1 broccoli head, florets separated

Salt and black pepper to the taste

2 garlic cloves, minced

2 bacon slices, chopped

2 tablespoons ghee

Directions:

1. Heat up a pot with the ghee over medium high heat, add garlic and bacon, stir and cook for 3 minutes.

2. Add cauliflower and broccoli florets, stir and cook for 2 minutes more.

3. Add water to cover them, cover pot and simmer for 10 minutes.

4. Add salt and pepper, stir again and blend soup using an immersion blender.

5. Simmer for a couple more minutes over medium heat, ladle into bowls and serve.

Enjoy!

Nutrition: calories 230, fat 3, fiber 3, carbs 6, protein 10

Broccoli Stew

This veggie stew is just delicious!

Preparation time: 10 minutes **Cooking time:** 40 minutes **Servings:** 4
Ingredients:

1 broccoli head, florets separated

2 teaspoons coriander seeds

A drizzle of olive oil

1 yellow onion, chopped

Salt and black pepper to the taste

A pinch of red pepper, crushed

1 small ginger piece, chopped

1 garlic clove, minced

28 ounces canned tomatoes, pureed

Directions:

1. Put water in a pot, add salt, bring to a boil over medium high heat, add broccoli florets, steam them for 2 minutes, transfer them to a bowl filled with ice water, drain them and leave aside.

2. Heat up a pan over medium high heat, add coriander seeds, toast them for 4 minutes, transfer to a grinder, ground them and leave aside as well.

3. Heat up a pot with the oil over medium heat, add onions, salt, pepper and red pepper, stir and cook for 7 minutes.

4. Add ginger, garlic and coriander seeds, stir and cook for 3 minutes.

5. Add tomatoes, bring to a boil and simmer for 10 minutes.

6. Add broccoli, stir and cook your stew for 12 minutes.

7. Divide into bowls and serve.

Enjoy!

Nutrition: calories 150, fat 4, fiber 2, carbs 5, protein 12

Amazing Watercress Soup

A Chinese style keto soup sounds pretty amazing, doesn't it?

Preparation time: 10 minutes **Cooking time:** 10 minutes **Servings:** 4

Ingredients:

6 cup chicken stock

¼ cup sherry

2 teaspoons coconut aminos

6 and ½ cups watercress

Salt and black pepper to the taste

2 teaspoons sesame seed

3 shallots, chopped

3 egg whites, whisked

Directions:

1. Put stock into a pot, mix with salt, pepper, sherry and coconut aminos, stir and bring to a boil over medium high heat.

2. Add shallots, watercress and egg whites, stir, bring to a boil, divide into bowls and serve with sesame seeds sprinkled on top.

Enjoy!

Nutrition: calories 50, fat 1, fiber 0, carbs 1, protein 5

Delicious Bok Choy Soup

You can even have this for dinner!

Preparation time: 10 minutes **Cooking time:** 15 minutes **Servings:** 4

Ingredients:

3 cups beef stock

1 yellow onion, chopped

1 bunch bok choy, chopped

1 and ½ cups mushrooms, chopped

Salt and black pepper to the taste

½ tablespoon red pepper flakes

3 tablespoons coconut aminos

3 tablespoons parmesan, grated

2 tablespoons Worcestershire sauce

2 bacon strips, chopped

Directions:

1. Heat up a pot over medium high heat, add bacon, stir, cook until it until it's crispy, transfer to paper towels and drain grease.

2. Heat up the pot again over medium heat, add mushrooms and onions, stir and cook for 5 minutes.

3. Add stock, bok choy, coconut aminos, salt, pepper, pepper flakes and Worcestershire sauce, stir, cover and cook until bok choy is tender.

4. Ladle soup into bowls, sprinkle parmesan and bacon and serve. Enjoy!

Nutrition: calories 100, fat 3, fiber 1, carbs 2, protein 6

Bok Choy Stir Fry

It's simple, it's easy and very delicious!

Preparation time: 10 minutes **Cooking time:** 7 minutes **Servings:** 2

Ingredients:

2 garlic cloves, minced

2 cup bok choy, chopped

2 bacon slices, chopped

Salt and black pepper to the taste

A drizzle of avocado oil

Directions:

1. Heat up a pan with the oil over medium heat, add bacon, stir and brown until it's crispy, transfer to paper towels and drain grease.

2. Return pan to medium heat, add garlic and bok choy, stir and cook for 4 minutes.

3. Add salt, pepper and return bacon, stir, cook for 1 minute more, divide between plates and serve.

Enjoy!

Nutrition: calories 50, fat 1, fiber 1, carbs 2, protein 2

Cream Of Celery

This will impress you!

Preparation time: 10 minutes **Cooking time:** 40 minutes **Servings:** 4

Ingredients:

1 bunch celery, chopped

Salt and black pepper to the taste

3 bay leaves

½ garlic head, chopped

2 yellow onions, chopped

4 cups chicken stock

¾ cup heavy cream

2 tablespoons ghee

Directions:

1. Heat up a pot with the ghee over medium high heat, add onions, salt and pepper, stir and cook for 5 minutes.

2. Add bay leaves, garlic and celery, stir and cook for 15 minutes.

3. Add stock, more salt and pepper, stir, cover pot, reduce heat and simmer for 20 minutes.

4. Add cream, stir and blend everything using an immersion blender.

5. Ladle into soup bowls and serve.

Enjoy!

Nutrition: calories 150, fat 3, fiber 1, carbs 2, protein 6

Delightful Celery Soup

It's so delightful and delicious! Try it!

Preparation time: 10 minutes **Cooking time:** 25 minutes **Servings:** 8

Ingredients:

26 ounces celery leaves and stalks, chopped

1 tablespoon onion flakes

Salt and black pepper to the taste

3 teaspoons fenugreek powder

3 teaspoons veggie stock powder

10 ounces sour cream

Directions:

1. Put celery into a pot, add water to cover, add onion flakes, salt, pepper, stock powder and fenugreek powder, stir, bring to a boil over medium heat and simmer for 20 minutes.

2. Use an immersion blender to make your cream, add sour cream, more salt and pepper and blend again.

3. Heat up soup again over medium heat, ladle into bowls and serve.

Enjoy!

Nutrition: calories 140, fat 2, fiber 1, carbs 5, protein 10

Amazing Celery Stew

This Iranian style keto stew is so tasty and easy to make!

Preparation time: 10 minutes **Cooking time:** 30 minutes **Servings:** 6

Ingredients:

1 celery bunch, roughly chopped

1 yellow onion, chopped

1 bunch green onion, chopped

4 garlic cloves, minced

Salt and black pepper to the taste

1 parsley bunch, chopped

2 mint bunches, chopped

3 dried Persian lemons, pricked with a fork

2 cups water

2 teaspoons chicken bouillon

4 tablespoons olive oil

Directions:

1. Heat up a pot with the oil over medium high heat, add onion, green onions and garlic, stir and cook for 6 minutes.

2. Add celery, Persian lemons, chicken bouillon, salt, pepper and water, stir, cover pot and simmer on medium heat for 20 minutes.

3. Add parsley and mint, stir and cook for 10 minutes more.

4. Divide into bowls and serve.

Enjoy!

Nutrition: calories 170, fat 7, fiber 4, carbs 6, protein 10

Spinach Soup

It's a textured and creamy keto soup you have to try soon!

Preparation time: 10 minutes **Cooking time:** 15 minutes **Servings:** 8

Ingredients:

2 tablespoons ghee

20 ounces spinach, chopped

1 teaspoon garlic, minced

Salt and black pepper to the taste

45 ounces chicken stock

½ teaspoon nutmeg, ground

2 cups heavy cream

1 yellow onion, chopped

Directions:

1. Heat up a pot with the ghee over medium heat, add onion, stir and cook for 4 minutes.

2. Add garlic, stir and cook for 1 minute.

3. Add spinach and stock, stir and cook for 5 minutes.

4. Blend soup with an immersion blender and heat up the soup again.

5. Add salt, pepper, nutmeg and cream, stir and cook for 5 minutes more.

6. Ladle into bowls and serve.

Enjoy!

Nutrition: calories 245, fat 24, fiber 3, carbs 4, protein 6

Delicious Mustard Greens Sauté

This is so tasty!

Preparation time: 10 minutes **Cooking time:** 20 minutes **Servings:** 4

Ingredients:

2 garlic cloves, minced

1 tablespoon olive oil

2 and ½ pounds collard greens, chopped

1 teaspoon lemon juice

1 tablespoon ghee

Salt and black pepper to the taste

Directions:

1. Put some water in a pot, add salt and bring to a simmer over medium heat.

2. Add greens, cover and cook for 15 minutes.

3. Drain collard greens well, press out liquid and put them into a bowl.

4. Heat up a pan with the oil and the ghee over medium high heat, add collard greens, salt, pepper and garlic.

5. Stir well and cook for 5 minutes.

6. Add more salt and pepper if needed, drizzle lemon juice, stir, divide between plates and serve.

Enjoy!

Nutrition: calories 151, fat 6, fiber 3, carbs 7, protein 8

CPSIA information can be obtained
at www.ICGtesting.com
Printed in the USA
BVHW052302260421
605864BV00007B/1571

9 781802 220056